SUMMER BODY

BIGGER LEANER STRONGER

PIERRE – OLIVIER JOYAL

Disclaimer & Legal Notice

"Exactly 1 year ago, I was working like a madman, I was only feeling successful professionally. I started working out with no specific goals in mind, I only had the motivation to start, but you found exactly what I needed. You helped me transform myself physically and mentally. I'm lucky to have you as a coach, you have remained human and very encouraging throughout the process"

- **Trèflé M**

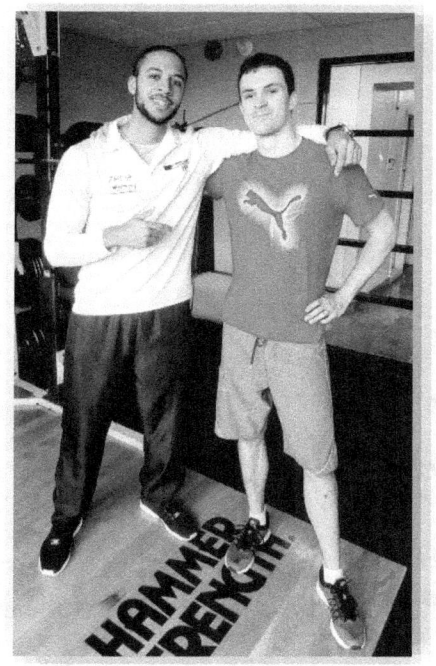

https://vimeo.com/335250812

"When I started working out with you, I was 235 (lb). You were the 1st person I met at the gym. I was scared because I previously tried to lose weight by myself and it did not work. People like you are rare because you are so human, you pushed me to become a better person every day. Now I am 180 (lb), I'm a lot lighter, I love myself even more than before and I have more energy. Honestly, my life changed and I'm happy I have met you."

- David B.

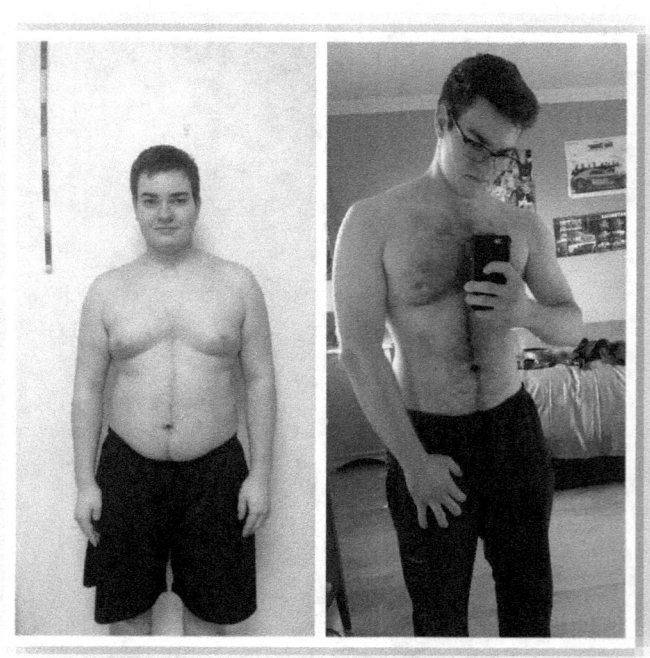

https://vimeo.com/345389271

TABLE OF CONTENT

Why You Should Listen To Pierre-Olivier?

Pierre-Olivier received his Master's Degree in Physical Therapy from McGill University. He played high school and college basketball at a high level and developed the skill set to serve these type of athletes. After his basketball career, he started personal training with clients one on one and his mission is to make everyone to be in a state of complete physical, mental and social well being.

Pierre-Olivier also possesses an extensive knowledge of nutrition that he has simplified for the masses and both practices and preaches with outstanding results.

YOUR FIRST DAY AT THE GYM

Assess Body Composition

- Take pictures of yourself from the front, side and back (every 6 weeks).

- Measure your bodyweight in lb (every week) and body fat % (every 4 weeks), if you have a bioelectrical machine.

- Measure your waist circumference (every 2 weeks), arms size, legs if important.

Assess Strength

Your upper and lower body strength is measured by determining 1 rep max on your squat and bench press. The 1-rep max is the most weight you can lift once for an exercise. It will be used to find out how much weight you should lift in other repetition ranges. Find your (1RM) for bench press & squats using this formula.

- Warm up sets (to wake up your nervous system, the goal is not to fatigue your muscles).

  - Lift the bar X 10 reps.

  - Lift a lightweight X 5 reps.

  - Lift a moderate weight X 3 reps.

  - Lift a heavyweight X 1 reps (then rest for 2-5 min).

- Attempt to your 1st of 3 attempts to measure your 1- rep max and use a spotter for bench press and a power rack for squats.

Example:

Warm-up sets

- #1 Barbell (45 lb) / 45 lb X 10 reps

- #2 Barbell + 2 X (10 lb) / 65 lb X 5 reps

- #3 Barbell + 2 X (25 lb) / 95 lb X 3 reps

- #4 Barbell + 2 X (35 lb) / 115 lb X 1 rep

1 Rep Max Attempt

- #1 Barbell + 2 X (45 lb) / 135 lb X 1 rep

- #2 Barbell + 2 X (50 lb) / 145 lb X 1 rep

- #3 Barbell + 2 X (55 lb) / 155 lb X 1 rep

If you don't feel comfortable with your squat technique, go see a personal trainer/physiotherapist to improve your technique. Learn how to squat watching this video. Replace Squat with Leg Press.

https://youtu.be/VUS8lcYcuu4

BENCH PRESS and **SQUATS** will be the main exercise of your summer body workout for the upper & lower body.

Assess Cardio

It is very important to measure your aerobic capacity. If you consider yourself a beginner, do the **12 min run test**. If you consider yourself an intermediate or advanced runner, do the **1.5 miles Cooper Test**.

How to perform the 12 min run test?

- Hop on the treadmill and run or walk as far as possible in a 12 minutes period. Try to cover the maximum distance. The incline must stay at 0. Keep track of how much distance you covered. Normally, it varies around 1.2 & 2.2 km in 12 minutes.

How to perform the 1.5 miles / 2.4 km Cooper Test?

- This run test is a simple running test of aerobic fitness. Hop on the treadmill and run (1.5 miles / 2.4 km) with the incline at 0. Finish the distance as fast as possible. I can do it in 9:34 min.

Other Strength / Endurance Test

Max Chin Up & Max Dips Test:

Perform as many repetitions as you can in a row. If you can't do one, use the elastic to help support your body weight. Only count repetition that covers the full range of motion.

The final step is to write all of your results of the evaluation in your training log. (Bodyweight, Picture taken, Waist (cm), 1 Rep Max Bench Press (lb), 1 Rep Max Squat (lb), Max Chin Up (reps),

Max Dips (reps), Cardio 12 min (distance covered) or 1.5 miles (time).

Click the link below to see the video explanation of what you must do your first day at the gym!

https://youtu.be/TlVC8EtbkXo

Goals

Warning: *If you work out consistently for 4 days/week, improve your nutritional habits and use a training/nutrition log for 12 weeks you will…*

If your body fat is above 12% you must prioritize to lose weight, expect to;

- Lose 0.3-0.5 body fat % / week = (1.2-2%/month).

- Lose 0.3-0.5 cm waist circumference / week = (1.2-2cm/month).

- Lose 1-2 (lb) of body fat / week = (4-8 lb/month)

If your body fat is at or below 12% you can prioritize gaining weight & muscle, expect to;

- Gain 1-2 (lb) of lean muscle/month if you eat in a caloric surplus (your bodyweight (lb) X 18-20).

- Increase your 1 rep max bench press by 20-30 lb in 12 weeks.

- Increase your 1 rep max squat by 30 lb and more in 12 weeks.

If you are overweight/obese you can aim to lose 10 % of your current bodyweight in six (6) months.

Ex: Body Mass Index >30, Man Height 5'10 weighting 210 lb

Bodyweight 210 lb X 90% = 190 lb in (6) months.

Click the link below have more information about goal setting!

https://youtu.be/sf8w6xdr9oY

Should I bulk or cut first?

If your body fat percentage is above 12%, aim to cut first. When you are at 12% or when you can see your abs in the mirror you can decide to bulk up or keep cutting.

UPPER & LOWER BODY WORKOUT PLAN

TRAINING SCHEDULE

Day	Workout
Monday	Upper Body
Tuesday	Lower Body
Wednesday	Off (Abs & Cardio)
Thursday	Upper Body
Friday	Lower Body
Saturday	Off (Abs & Cardio)
Sunday	Off

CARDIO PROTOCOL

"If you have **more than 20 lb** of fat to lose, add cardio and abs Wednesday and Saturday"

UPPER BODY WORKOUT WEEK 1-4

Order	Exercise	Sets	Reps	Tempo	Rest
1	Bench Press	4	8	3-0-2	90 secs
2	Incline Barbell Press	3	10	3-0-2	60 secs
3	Lat Pull Down	3	10	3-0-2	60 secs
4	Seated Cable Row	3	10	3-0-2	60 secs
5A	Cable Biceps Curls	3	10-12	3-0-2	*
5B	Cable Triceps Extension	3	10-12	3-0-2	60 secs

Cardio	Phases		Duration	Speed	Intensity	Total
Treadmill	4X	1st	2 min	10 km/h	Moderate (Jog)	12 min
Week 1-4		2nd	1 min	13 km/h	Intense (Run)	

	Abs Tabata				Total
Exercise	Toe Touch	Leg Raises	Roman Twist	V-Crunch	4 min
Duration	20-sec work & 10-sec rest for each exercise				

8

LOWER BODY WORKOUT WEEK 1-4

Order	Exercise	Sets	Reps	Tempo	Rest
1	Squat	4	8	3-0-2	90 secs
2	Leg Curl	3	10	3-0-2	60 secs
3	Leg Extension	3	10	3-0-2	60 secs
4	Lumbar Extension	3	10	3-0-2	60 secs
5	Standing Calf Raises	3	10-12	3-0-2	60 secs

Cardio	Phases		Duration	Speed	Intensity	Total
Bike	4X	1st	2 min	80 RPM	Moderate (Level 10)	12 min
Week 1-4		2nd	1 min	110 RPM	Intense (Level 14)	

Abs Tabata					Total
Exercise	Plank	Side Plank	Side Plank	Mountain Climbers	4 min
Duration	20-sec work & 10-sec rest for each exercise				

9

UPPER BODY WORKOUT WEEK 5-8

Order	Exercise	Sets	Reps	Tempo	Rest
1	Bench Press	4	5	4-0-2	90 secs
2	Incline Barbell Press	3	8	4-0-2	60 secs
3	Lat Pull Down	3	8	4-0-2	60 secs
4	Seated Cable Row	3	8	4-0-2	60 secs
5A	Cable Biceps Curls	3	8-10	4-0-2	*
5B	Cable Triceps Extension	3	8-10	4-0-2	60 secs

Cardio	Phases		Duration	Speed	Intensity	Total
Treadmill	4X	1st	**1 m 30**	10 km/h	Moderate (Jog)	12 min
Week 5-8		2nd	**1 m 30**	13 km/h	Intense (Run)	

Abs Tabata					Total
Exercise	Toe Touch	Leg Raises	Roman Twist	V-Crunch	5 : 20
Duration	**30-sec work & 10-sec rest** for each exercise				

LOWER BODY WORKOUT WEEK 5-8

Order	Exercise	Sets	Reps	Tempo	Rest
1	Squat	4	5	4-0-2	90 secs
2	Leg Curl	3	8	4-0-2	60 secs
3	Leg Extension	3	8	4-0-2	60 secs
4	Lumbar Extension	3	8	4-0-2	60 secs
5	Standing Calf Raises	3	8-10	4-0-2	60 secs

Cardio	Phases		Duration	Speed	Intensity	Total
Bike	4X	1st	1 m 30	80 RPM	Moderate (Level 10)	12 min
Week 5-8		2nd	1 m 30	110 RPM	Intense (Level 14)	

	Abs Tabata				Total
Exercise	Plank	Side Plank	Side Plank	Mountain Climbers	5: 20
Duration	**30-sec work & 10-sec rest** for each exercise				

11

UPPER BODY WORKOUT WEEK 9-11

Order	Exercise	Sets	Reps	Tempo	Rest
1	Bench Press	4	3	5-0-1	90 secs
2	Incline Barbell Press	3	6	5-0-1	60 secs
3	Lat Pull Down	3	6	5-0-1	60 secs
4	Seated Cable Row	3	6	5-0-1	60 secs
5A	Cable Biceps Curls	3	6-8	5-0-1	*
5B	Cable Triceps Extension	3	6-8	5-0-1	60 secs

Cardio	Phases		Duration	Speed	Intensity	Total
Treadmill	4X	1st	1 min	10 km/h	Moderate (Jog)	12 min
Week 9-11		2nd	2 min	13 km/h	Intense (Run)	

	Abs Tabata				Total
Exercise	Toe Touch	Leg Raises	Roman Twist	V-Crunch	6 : 40
Duration	**40-sec work & 10-sec rest** for each exercise				

LOWER BODY WORKOUT WEEK 9-11

Order	Exercise	Sets	Reps	Tempo	Rest
1	Squat	4	3	5-0-1	90 secs
2	Leg Curl	3	6	5-0-1	60 secs
3	Leg Extension	3	6	5-0-1	60 secs
4	Lumbar Extension	3	6	5-0-1	60 secs
5	Standing Calf Raises	3	6-8	5-0-1	60 secs

Cardio	Phases		Duration	Speed	Intensity	Total
Bike	4X	1st	**1 min**	80 RPM	Moderate (Level 10)	12 min
Week 9-11		2nd	**2 min**	110 RPM	Intense (Level 14)	

	Abs Tabata				Total
Exercise	Plank	Side Plank	Side Plank	Mountain Climbers	6: 40
Duration	**40-sec work & 10-sec rest** for each exercise				

13

BENCH PRESS &
SQUAT PROGRESSION

Week	Sets	Reps	Intensity	Ex: 1 Rep Max = 200 lb
1	4	8	72,5	145
2	4	8	75	150
3	4	8	77,5	155
4	4	8	80	160
5	4	5	82,5	165
6	4	5	85	170
7	4	5	87,5	175
8	4	5	90	180
9	4	3	92,5	185
10	4	3	95	190
11	4	3	97,5	195
12			Reassess your Strength 1 RM Bench Press & Squat	

INTENSITY

- Aim to add (5 lb = 2x 2.5 lb) to your Bench Press every week.
- Aim to add (10 lb = 2 x 5 lb) to your Squat every week.

How To Make It Work?

- If you miss one workout during the week, make sure to execute the workout missed during the same week.
- At your 12th week, re-assess your body composition, strength, and cardio.
- If you don't feel comfortable with your SQUAT technique, replace it the LEG PRESS MACHINE
- At your second upper and lower body workout of the week, you must go for a MAX REPS SETS for the last sets of every exercise. Why? Because it allows you to make sure the WEIGHT you are lifting is INTENSE enough for you.

    o Ex: Bench Press Set 1 – 8 reps, Set 2 – 8 reps, Set 3 8 reps, Set 4 MAX REPS SET 11 reps!

When Is It Time To Increase The Weight?

- Use the **rule of 2** " If you can successfully complete 2 or more repetition in the last set in two (2) consecutive workouts for any given exercise, then the load should be increased

NUTRITION STRATEGIES

#1 CARBS CYCLING

Carbs cycling is a nutritionally advanced method that can boost your muscle gain and fat loss process for a short duration. It is a strategy where you eat less carbs on days when your rest or do light intensity cardio workouts, and on your resistance training days, you eat more carbs.

In order to understand how it works, you must know what insulin is and how to use it to your advantage. Insulin is a hormone that helps to promote the building of muscle mass or the accumulation of fat. Its main job is to maintain a safe and steady blood glucose level of around **80-100 (mg/dl.)**

When blood glucose level rises above 100, the pancreas secretes insulin and then the hormone takes the extra glucose out of the blood and takes it to storage.

There are 3 different storage depots for extra glucose:

- Muscle glycogen.
- Liver glycogen.
- Fat cells (Not good!).

Of course, we prefer glucose to be stored in our muscle. However, insulin does not care about your fitness goals, it simply regulates.

The GOOD side of insulin is that it builds muscle, it stops the breakdown of muscle (inhibit catabolism of protein) and it transports amino acid into muscle cells.

The BAD side of insulin is that it promotes glucose transport into the fat cell, it decreases the use of fat (put that in another way, insulin "spares fat") and it increases fatty acid synthesis in the liver, which is not good for your body composition and that is how most people become fat.

How to use it to your advantage?

Insulin is simply an anabolic transport hormone that does its job and does not care whether you gain fat or gain muscle. It only cares about keeping blood glucose in the normal range. When blood glucose rises above normal, insulin will be secreted and will quickly restore normal glucose level.

It is not the function of insulin to secrete itself at the right time, it's up to YOU to stimulate insulin release at the right time, and there is a way to do that.

Want to gain muscle?

If your primary goal is to gain muscle, you want higher levels of insulin throughout the day. Also, you especially want the high insulin level after training, so eat carbs dense food post workout.

Want to lose fat?

If your goal is strictly fat loss, then you want lower levels of insulin throughout the day. You do it by eating meals that consist mainly of **proteins and vegetables**.

Even if you don't care about gaining muscle mass, it is still important to initiate insulin secretion post-workout. This will stop the breakdown of muscle cells. Otherwise, you'll find yourself losing valuable muscle.

Want to gain muscle AND lose fat at the same time?

You cannot burn fat and build muscle at the EXACT SAME TIME, but you can do both on the same day.

When blood glucose is high, insulin is secreted and glucose is stored in muscle glycogen or liver glycogen. When blood glucose is low, insulin secretion is diminished and fat becomes the body's primary fuel source. You can plan your day to have periods of time focused on building muscle and periods of time focused on burning fat. If you want to gain muscle faster, increase the amount of insulin you secrete especially immediately after resistance training. Why? Because insulin will not convert glucose to fat if it can first store it as glycogen. Thus, after an intense weight training session, both muscle and liver glycogen are depleted and ready to soak up serious glucose. So, **don't be shy with the carbs post workout!**

Watch this for a video explanation!
https://youtu.be/gjXs27-OF6k

#2 COUNTING CALORIES

To burn fat, you have to be in a caloric deficit. How can you be in a caloric deficit? Take your body weight in (lb) and multiply that by 10-12 to gain weight, multiply by 18-20 to maintain, and also multiply by 14-16

Watch me explain it in this video!

https://youtu.be/Bteyyn-1PDU

Example: 200 lb man that want to

- **lose** weight

200 lb X (10-12) = 2000-2400 calories / day

- **maintain** weight

200 lb X (14-16) = 2800-3200 calories / day

- **gain** weight

200 lb X (18-20) = 3600-4000 calories / day

However, I'm sure you don't even know how many calories you are eating a day, unless you are a professional body-builder. So, your biggest problem now is that you are not aware of how much food you are eating. You spend too much time looking at what you SHOULD eat, but not enough time looking at what you

ARE eating now. Stop this bad habit and start being aware of what you are putting inside your one and only body.

Step 1 Awareness

- Use the free application *My Fitness Pal* available in iPhone and Android and keep track of everything that you are eating for 2 days of the week and one day of the weekend.

Learn how to become aware of your nutrition clicking the link below.

https://youtu.be/yhBGh3iWGiI

Step 2 Analysis

- Calculate your estimated caloric intake with the formula I presented above and analyze if you are eating a quantity of food that will force your body to change consistently.

Step 3 Action

- Copy a meal plan that will allow you to consume your desired amount of calories per day and do it consistently for 2 weeks.

Step 4 Adjust

- After adhering with your meal plan by weighing, and measuring everything you eat re-assess your body weight and body composition and adjust your nutritional habits.

The problem with counting calories is that you will not do it consistently. I've been training people for six (6) years, and there is only a small percentage of people like professional body-builders that are able to do it consistently. And if you are a professional fitness elite you are not only getting advice from an eBook! The only way to accurately count calories is by preparing and weighing everything you eat and store it inside of many containers.

That is why I use a better and efficient method called the **Portion Size Method**

#3 PORTION SIZE METHOD

Let's get one thing straight; I did NOT invent the portion size method. I've read multiple books in the subject of fitness and the company's Precision Nutrition explained it very well.

Instead of counting calories, you use "portion size", all you need is your own hand. A portion is the size of your **OPEN HAND** or **CLOSED FIST**. Here is how it works.

- Your palm determines your protein portions.
- Your closed fist determines your veggie portions.
- Your cupped hand determines your carbs portions.

(Credit goes to Precision Nutrition's, Forget Calorie Counting article for the following pictures and descriptions.)

Watch me give brief explanation about the portion size method. https://youtu.be/Qlq6kElKxXE

How To Determine Your Protein Intake?

Eat protein-dense foods like meat, fish, eggs, dairy or beans and use a palm-sized serving. A palm-size portion is the same thickness and diameter as your palm.

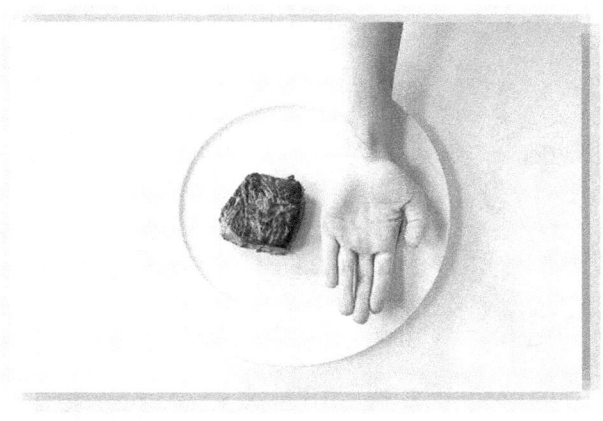

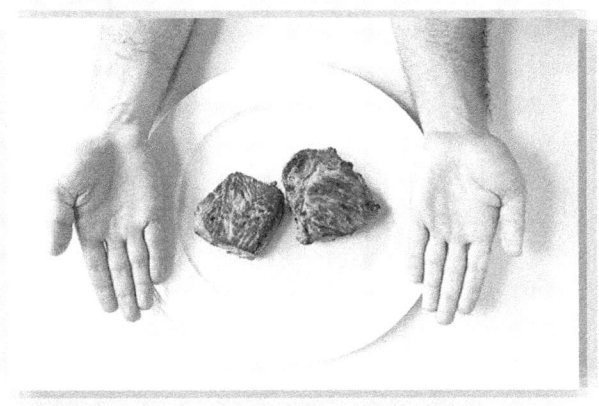

How To Determine Your Vegetable Intake?

For vegetable like carrots, broccoli, spinach, salad, etc. use a fist-sized serving.

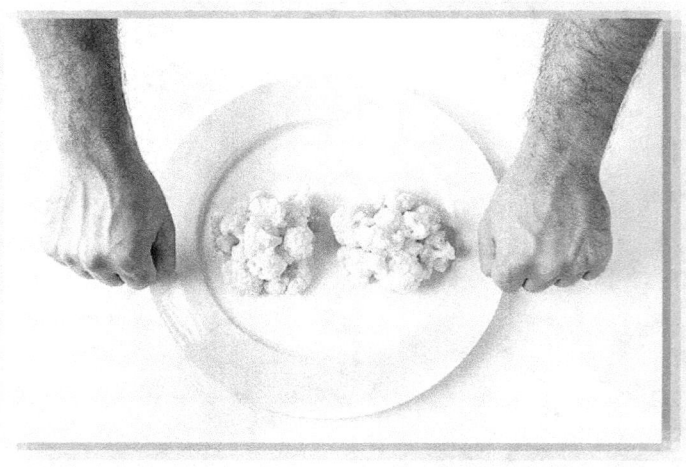

How To Determine Your Carbs Intake?

For your carbs like rice, potatoes, fruits, etc. use the palm of your cupped hand.

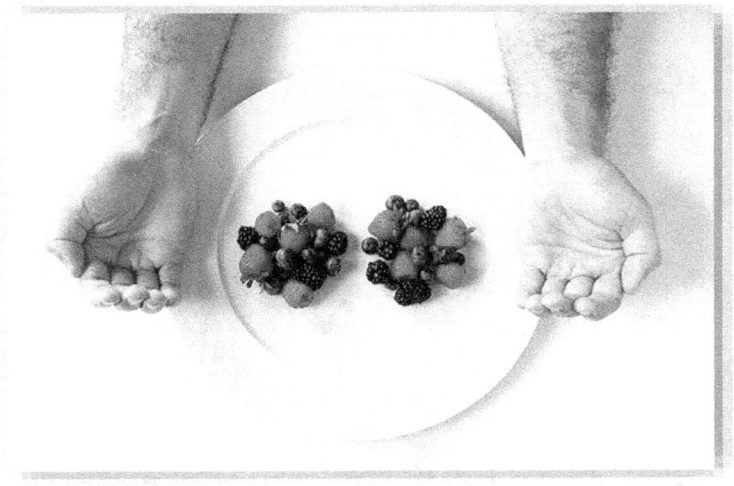

The Portion Size Method For Fat Loss

To lose bodyweight, you'll want to start with 1 portion of lean meat and 1-2 portions or green, leafy vegetable. You then have 1-2 cupped hand size of carbs POST WORKOUT ONLY!

You can eat that all day and eat as many meals as you want, as long as you keep your protein to one portion size and that is to keep your insulin levels low.

Now it is very important to keep track of everything. I've been having the best results of my life doing it. In this video, I show you how I keep track of everything. Start by committing to keep track of everything for 12 weeks.

When I have big goals I keep track of

- Everything I eat and drink, at what time I eat it, in a way that I can understand myself
- Every training, every reps, set, how much rest between sets,
- How many hours I sleep
- My mood to be aware of what makes me feel good, bad, etc.

By keeping track of EVERYTHING you can easily see if you are making progress or not, but more importantly, you will know WHY you are making progress or not! Everybody I know who has achieved extreme success and its awesome shape keeps a detailed nutrition and fitness log. So if people that are in better shape than you are doing it, who are you to not keep track of your nutrition and workouts?

Click below to see how I keep track of everything!

https://youtu.be/cSideaxoipA

#4 INTERMITTENT FASTING

Do you really want to know how to lose 10 lb in 2 weeks?

That is called **intermittent fasting.** To learn more click below.

https://youtu.be/KOPvGqgB8hA

I've spent four (4) months consistently experimenting this tactic to burn fat and build muscle, and you will learn the benefits and drawback of using this method for burning fat. It is not a type of fast where you don't eat all day long. The method that I used is the one that I fast for 16h a day (including sleep) and I give myself feeding windows of 8h to eat everything. During my "fasting window" (time that I'm not supposed to eat), I can consume everything that does not contain calories like water, coffee or green tea. During my 8h of "feeding window," I keep good nutritional habits.

Exemples :

8: 00 Am	Wake up, 3-4 glass of water
1: 30 pm / Pre-Workout	10 grams of (BCAA)
3 :00 pm / Post-Workout	Meal #1
5: 00 pm	Meal #2
8: 00 pm	Meal #3
11: 00 pm	Meal #4

In the morning, you can skip breakfast and push your first meal to a later moment that day. Here is what it looks like to have a better idea.

Why is it so effective?

When you skip breakfast and push your first meal to a later moment that day, you can eat more food in less time. Accordingly, if your meals are bigger, you will feel satisfied for a longer period of time than if you would have tried to eat small meals all day long.

The effect of fasting when burning fat

Using this technique forces your body to use his main reserve of energy *(fat)* in order to function optimally. The clients that are very busy usually love this approach because skipping breakfast gives them time to do things like working.

Also, recent research has proven these benefits.

- **Trial fasting is a great way to practice managing hunger.**
- **More regular fasting makes it easier to maintain a lower body fat percentage.**
- **Intermittent fasting can work, but it's not for everyone.**

The negative effect of intermittent fasting

This useful method to accelerate fat loss can be very difficult to adhere to if you don't keep a water bottle with you at all time. Dealing with hunger is the toughest thing to manage during the 1st 2 weeks. Once your body and hormones get used to skipping breakfast, it becomes easy to burn fat. The main takeaway in intermittent fasting is one method you can experiment with for at least two (2) weeks, but this is not for everyone.

Best Protein Sources

Try to avoid anything fried

Recommended proteins:

- Lean meats: Ground beef, chicken, turkey
- Fish: Salmon, Tuna, Tilapia
- Eggs
- Milk-based: cottage cheese, Greek yogurt
- Beans, peas, legumes, tofu
- Protein supplement: Milk-based Whey, Casein, Plant-based: pea, rice soy

Best Carbohydrate Sources

If your goal is strictly fat loss, you should avoid carbohydrates in general because they have a high caloric load and they spike insulin levels.

Recommended carbohydrates:

- Complex carbs: Bread, pasta, corn, sweet potato, quinoa, rice
- Simple sugar (Eat occasionally): Desserts, Fruit juice, soda

Best Vegetable Sources

- Broccoli, snow peas, lettuce, spinach, cucumber, peppers, any green vegetable!

BONUS #1 ABS & CARDIO

Before we get into training your abs, it is important to clarify one thing. Many men and women think they can do abs exercises to burn the fat stored there, but that is not how it works.

You can't spot remove fat around the belly. You have to do it **cumulatively**. Even if you build the most impressive six-pack imaginable, if there's fat covering it, you won't be able to see it.

You should still train your abs, but to lose body fat, dieting and staying in a caloric deficit is critical.

How to train your abs depends on your goal. When gaining weight to build muscle mass, resistance training targeting your abs are more beneficial because they thicken the muscle, which helps the abs "pop". However, when you are losing body fat, use body weight exercises in a circuit fashion to increase your heart rate and expend energy.

If you want to burn fat, use the abs workouts shown in this program or create your own. Choose ONE lower abs exercise, ONE oblique exercise, and TWO total core exercises. Do the first exercise for 20 seconds, then rest for 10 seconds, then the next abs exercise for 20 seconds followed by another 10 seconds of rest and so on for all four exercises. Then repeat them all twice.

You can also go at the **Fit Men Labs YouTube Channel** and execute the workouts every other day.

ABS & CARDIO WORKOUT

****Warm Up adequately before performing each of these intense fat burning workout routines to minimize the risk of injury by jogging on the treadmill 5 min**

Go at https://youtu.be/msHHsPpuwy8
Fit Men Labs YouTube Channel And Watch the **Hollywood Abs & Cardio Playlist** and do the 6 abs & cardio workout!

AMRAP stands for "as many rounds as possible." It's a workout structure frequently used for conditioning that pushes your body to the max within a set period of time. You will do it for 4 min.

1.   4 mins **AMRAP Workout 1**

AMRAP #1 :

20 Lunges

40 Jump Rope

20 Jumping Jack

40 High Knees

2.   4 min **AMRAP Workout 2**

AMRAP #2 :

25 Ski Jumps

20 Sumo Squats

15 Power Jacks

10 Push Ups

5 Burpees

3.   4 min **TABATA Abs Workout 1**

Round 1:

** 10 seconds rest between exercises

Step Up – 20 seconds

Low Jumping Jacks – 20 seconds

Tuck Jumps – 20 seconds

Ski Jump – 20 seconds

Round 2:

** 10 seconds rest between exercises

Step Up – 20 seconds

Low Jumping Jacks – 20 seconds

Tuck Jumps – 20 seconds

Ski Jump – 20 seconds

4.   4 min **TABATA Abs Workout 2**

Round 1:

** 10 seconds rest between exercises

Toe Touches – 20 seconds

Leg Raises – 20 seconds

Roman Twist – 20 seconds

V Crunch – 20 seconds

Round 2:

** 10 seconds rest between exercises

Toe Touches – 20 seconds

Leg Raises – 20 seconds

Roman Twist – 20 seconds

V Crunch – 20 seconds

5.   4 min Interval Cardio Workout 1

Round 1:

** 10 seconds rest between exercises

Jump Lunges – 50 seconds

High Knees – 50 seconds

Push Ups – 50 seconds

In & Out – 50 seconds

6.   4 min Tabata Abs Workout 3

Round 1:

** 10 seconds rest between exercises

V-Sit – 20 seconds

V- Crunch – 20 seconds

Hip Raises – 20 seconds

Side Plank Left – 20 seconds

Side Plank Right – 20 seconds

Toe Touches – 20 seconds

Roman Twist – 20 seconds

Bicycles – 20 seconds

BONUS #2 SLEEP

One of the easiest ways to burn fat and build muscle is to simply get more sleep. Those who sleep less (5h30) lose more muscle than those who sleep more (8h30). People that are sleep deprived produce more of the appetite-stimulating hormone ghrelin. As a result, they wake up hungrier.

When you lift weight, you are tearing the muscle in a healthy way. After you eat your body uses proteins to repair your muscle. However, your body will not start repairing your muscle until you are at rest for an extended period of time, such as sleep. So if you don't sleep enough, your body will not get enough time to repair and fully recover. So, make sure you're getting 7h-8h30 of sleep each night. You will feel better, and be much stronger. And like everything else, keep track of your sleep by nothing what time you fall asleep and what time you wake.

Pre-workouts can be good if you want more energy. However, don't forget to sleep.

BONUS #3 GROCERY LIST

Meat and dairy products

- ☐ Ground beef, 1-2 lb
- ☐ Chicken breast, 1-2 lb
- ☐ Turkey breast, 1-2 lb
- ☐ Salmon, 1 lb
- ☐ 3 Dozen eggs
- ☐ 1 Carton of yogurt
- ☐ A little bit of cheese

Fruits and vegetables

- ☐ Fresh spinach, 1 lb
- ☐ Mushroom, ½ lb
- ☐ Onion, 2 medium
- ☐ Tomatoes, 3 large
- ☐ Cucumber, 2 large
- ☐ Bell peppers, 2 medium
- ☐ Garlic, 1 clove
- ☐ Apple, 4
- ☐ Frozen blueberries, 1 bag
- ☐ Lemon, 4
- ☐ Fresh Berries (Strawberry, raspberry, blueberries) of your choice

Others

- ☐ Protein powder (2 lb)
- ☐ Chickpeas, 1-2 can
- ☐ Black beans, 1-2 can
- ☐ Oatmeal, 1 lb
- ☐ Quinoa, 1 lb
- ☐ Flaxseed, ½ lb
- ☐ Olive oil
- ☐ Butter or coconut oil
- ☐ Cooking spray
- ☐ Almond, 1lb
- ☐ Lemon juice, 1 bottle
- ☐ Salt and pepper
- ☐ Garlic powder
- ☐ Hot sauce
- ☐ Cinnamon
- ☐ Cumin
- ☐ Aluminum sheet
- ☐ Baking sheet

41

BONUS #4 MEAL PLANS

You learned that you should eat a palm of protein and a fist of vegetables with every meal and you may be wondering what this looks like on a meal-by-meal basis. With that in mind, Fit Men Labs created 3 sample meal plan for how this might look. We even provided estimated nutrition facts for you if you want to know your numbers. However, don't stress about counting calories and use the portion-sized method simply utilizing your hand.

Keep in mind the serving size depends on the size of your hand, your hunger and fullness cues, as well as your results.

Also, you'll notice that the fat loss examples have a cupped handful of carbs or a thumb of fats removed from some meals, and the muscle gain example have a cupped handful of carbs and/or a thumb of fats added to some meals.

1st Step
Follow this plan consistently for a few weeks

It typically takes between 2 and 4 weeks to determine whether a nutrition or exercise intervention is working. Consistency during this time is important to do your best.

2nd Step
Assess your progress regularly during this time

Based on your goals, monitor a number of indicators such as body weight, waist circumference, pictures and strength/performance measure regularly.

3rd Step
Make changes when necessary

If you want to **lose weight**, you'll need to cut back on a few portions. The easiest way is to cut out a handful of carbs or thumbs of fats from a few meals each day. It will have you eating about 250 fewer calories per day. Also, you'll need to eat SLOWLY.

However, if you want to **gain weight** you'll probably need to increase a few portion sizes. The easiest way is to add a 1-cupped handful of carbs or a thumb of fats to a few meals each day. It will have you eating about 250 more calories per day. Also, you'll need to eat FAST.

Equipment if you count calories (food scale, cups, and teaspoons)

Man looking to lose body weight and burn fat

BREAKFAST	2 palms of whole eggs (4 eggs) 2 fists of peppers and onions (2 cups) 1 cupped handful of oatmeal (2/3 cup) 1 cupped handful of berries (2/3 cup) 1 thumb of almonds (1 tbsp) water / green tea / black coffee
LUNCH	2 palms of chicken (200g) 2 fists of carrots (2 cups) 1 cupped handful of beans (2/3 cup) 2 thumbs of peanuts (2 tbsp) water / green tea / black coffee
POST WORKOUT SHAKE	2 scoops of chocolate protein 1 fist of spinach (1 cup) 1 cupped handful of berries (2/3 cup) 2 thumbs of almonds (2 tbsp) ice cubes as desired
DINNER	2 palms of salmon (225g) 2 fists of zucchini (2 cups) 1 cupped handful of sweet potato (1 medium) 1 thumb of extra virgin olive oil (1 tbsp) 1 thumb of butter (1 1bsp) water
ESTIMATED NUTRITION FACTS	**Protein :** 210 g (36%) **Carbs :** 165 g (28%) **Fats :** 95 g (36%) **Calories :** 2355

Man looking to improve health and body composition

BREAKFAST	2 palms of whole eggs (4 eggs) 2 fists portion of broccoli (2 cups) 1 cupped handful of oatmeal (2/3 cup) 1 cupped handful of berries (2/3 cup) 2 thumbs of almonds (2 tbsp) water / green tea / black coffee
LUNCH	2 palms of chicken (200 g) 2 fists of peppers and onions (2 cups) 1 cupped handful of beans (2/3 cup) 2 thumbs of guacamole (2 tbsp) water / green tea / black coffee
POST WORKOUT SHAKE	2 scoops of vanilla whey protein 1 cupped handful of frozen strawberries (2/3 cup) 1 cupped handful of banana (1 medium) 2 thumbs of walnuts (3 tbsp) 250 ml of milk/water/ or almond milk ice cubes as desired
DINNER	2 palms of salmon (225g) 2 fists of asparagus (2 cups) 2 cupped handfuls of potato (1 large) 1 thumb of extra virgin olive oil (1 tbsp) 1 thumb of butter (1 tbsp) water
ESTIMATED NUTRITION FACTS	**Protein :** 230 g (33%) **Carbs :** 250 g (36%) **Fats :** 95 g (31%) **Calories :** 2775

Man looking to gain weight and build muscle

BREAKFAST	2 palms of whole eggs (4 eggs)
	1 palm of-of chicken sausage (1 sausage)
	2 fist portion of spinach (2 cups)
	2 cupped handfuls of grain toast (2 slices)
	1 cupped handful of banana (1 medium)
	2 thumbs of peanut butter (2 thumbs)
	water / green tea / black coffee / juice

LUNCH	2 palms of chicken (200g)
	2 fists of mixed peppers and onions (2 cups)
	1 cupped handful of black beans (2/3 cup)
	2 cupped handfuls of rice (1 1/3 cups)
	2 thumbs of guacamole (2 tbsp)
	water / green tea / black coffee / juice

POST WORKOUT SHAKE	2 scoops of chocolate whey protein
	1 cupped handful of banana (1 medium)
	1 cupped handful of oatmeal (1 cup)
	3 thumbs of peanut butter (3 tbsp)
	250 ml of milk
	ice cubes as desired

DINNER	2 palms of salmon (225g)
	2 fists of zucchini (2 cups)
	1 cupped handful of sweet potato (1 medium)
	1 cupped handful of quinoa (1 1/3 cups)
	2 thumbs of extra virgin olive oil (2 tbsp)
	water/juice

ESTIMATED NUTRITION FACTS	**Protein :** 255 g (32%)
	Carbs : 295 g (36%)
	Fats : 115 g (32%)
	Calories : 3235

BONUS #5 SUPPLEMENTS

In the gym, a lot of guys are asking me "what supplements do you take?". There are a few supplements that I use to help me burn fat and build muscle. However, they are not more important than your nutritional habits. When it comes to eating healthy, understand that the quantity of food you are eating, the type of food you consume and understanding when to eat specific nutrients will have bigger impact in your physique than nutritional supplements. Now, let me share with you which one I recommend.

Whey Protein

Most of your dietary protein should come from meat, fish, poultry and eggs or plant-based whole foods if you are a plant-based eater. However, it is not always possible or practical particularly if you are busy or constantly on the go. In this case, a protein powder is what you want to investigate. Protein powder comes in many forms- whey, casein, milk protein blend, egg, soy, pea, rice are the most common.

You know that a whey protein is good for you if you are not farting after everytime you drink it. Ideally consume your shake with water if you want to lose weight or with milk if you try to gain weight. Also the whey protein must taste good.

Creatine

Creatine supplements is beneficial for good health as well as athletic performance. It has amazing regenerative effects on all tissues of the body I recommend you take 5 g per day, which amounts to about one teaspoon. That will increase your power output by about 10%. It means that in the gym, you will be able to lift much heavier loads and increase your athletic performance with explosive lifts.

I recommend you take a plain creatine monohydrate because most of the scientific research that has proven the benefits of this supplement was on regular creatine monohydrate, not the other ones.You don't need the never, fancier and more expensive creatine on the market.

Fish oil

Fish oil is rich in DHA and EPA, two powerful omega-3 fats responsible for things like decreased inflammation, increased metabolic rate, improved fat burning, increased carbohydrate storage in muscle, better glucose and insulin tolerance, reduced blood lipids. It increases thermogenesis, which is the number of calories that your body burn as heat energy each day. Fish oil also increase muscle anabolism (muscle growth), and decrease muscle catabolism (muscle breakdown).These are great reasons for bodybuilding purpose.

Vitamin D

Your body produces Vitamin D when your skin is exposed to sunlight. However, due to abundant use of sunscreens and indoor lifestyles, a large percentage of the population is deficient in this vitamin (especially if you have a dark skin and you live in a cold environment). Optimizing your vitamin D may decrease your risk of cancer, increase bone density, improve performance and body composition and even improve your mood..

THANK YOU

If you learn anything, give me a 5-star review on Amazon (if you bought it there!). Use the information in this book, don't simply read it.

If you don't take action 24h after reading this guide, you will never have the summer body of your dreams.

For more content Subscribe to

Fit Men Labs YouTube Channel

Thank you & dream big!

Pierre-Olivier Joyal
Personal Trainer/Physiotherapist